DISSOCIATED DIET 2025

120 Recipes Science and Innovation in Modern Nutrition, Food Strategies for a Healthy and Balanced Life

KLARLOCK

DISCLAIMER

This book aims to provide useful and informative material on the topics covered in the publication. It is sold with the understanding that the author and publisher are not engaged in rendering any personal medical, health care, or other professional services in the book. The reader should consult his or her physician, health care provider, or other competent professional before adopting any suggestions in this book or drawing any conclusions. The author and publisher expressly disclaim responsibility for any liability, loss, or risk, personal or otherwise, arising, directly or indirectly, from the use and application of any contents of this book.

NOTE

All the recipes in this book are designed for four people. For this quantity, the ingredients indicated in the recipes must be considered. If you need to change the portion, it is recommended to proportionally adjust the doses of the ingredients. It is also recommended to carefully follow the preparation and cooking instructions to obtain the best result. In the context of this book, when we refer to "a cup" as a unit of measurement for ingredients, we mean using a standard kitchen cup with a capacity of approximately 240 milliliters. It is essential to use a measuring cup to get the right quantities of ingredients. If you don't have a measuring cup, you can use a graduated measuring cup, making sure to correctly correspond to the proportions indicated. Here are some examples 1 Cup of flour 100 gr. 1 cup of rice 200 gr. 1 Cup of Quinoa 200 gr

RECIPES FIRST DISHES

95 WHOLE WHOLE RISOTTO WITH PORCINI MUSHROOMS

97 WHOLEWHEAT PENNE WITH TOMATOES AND OLIVES

99 LENTIL SOUP WITH CELERY AND CARROTS

101 CUCUMBER NOODLES WITH LEMON SAUCE

103 LIGHT ZUCCHINI AND RICOTTA LASAGNE

105 BASMATI RICE WITH GRILLED VEGETABLES

107 TOMATO SOUP WITH FRESH BASIL

109 CARROT SPAGHETTI WITH AVOCADO SAUCE

111 STEAM RAVIOLI WITH SPINACH AND RICOTTA

113 RISOTTO WITH SAFFRON AND ASPARAGUS

115 WHOLE FARFALLE WITH AUBERGINES AND TOMATOES

117 MINESTRONE WITH LEGUMES AND MIXED VEGETABLES

119 PENNE ALLA NORMA WITH AUBERGINES AND TOMATO

121 WILD RICE WITH MUSHROOMS AND PARSLEY

123 PEAS SOUP WITH FRESH MINT

125 PUMPKIN FETTUCCINE WITH PARSLEY PESTO

127 RICOTTA AND SPINACH RAVIOLI WITH TOMATO SAUCE

129 CUCUMBER SPAGHETTI WITH PRAWNS AND AVOCADO

131 LEMON RISOTTO WITH ASPARAGUS

133 PEARL BARLEY WITH TOMATOES AND ARUGULA

135 WHOLE WHOLE TAGLIATELLE WITH TOMATO SAUCE

137 CAULIFLOWER SOUP WITH TOASTED NUTS

139 PAPPARDELLE WITH LEAN MEAT SAUCE

RECIPES SECOND DISHES

212 DUCK BREAST WITH BLACK CURRANT SAUCE

214 COCONUT CHICKEN WITH WOKED VEGETABLES

216 BEEF STEAK WITH GREEN PEPPER

218 BAKED TROUT WITH ALMONDS

220 PORK FILLET WITH CRANBERRIES

222 CHICKEN WITH WALNUTS WITH ARUGULA SALAD

224 LAMB SHANK WITH MINT

225 SALMON IN PISTACHIO CRUST

227 VEAL CUTLETS MILANESE -STYLE

229 CHICKEN CURRY WITH SPINACH

231 BEEF STEAK WITH ROSEMARY

233 MEDITERRANEAN-STYLE COD

235 DUCK IN PLUM SAUCE

237 SWEET AND SOUR PORK WITH PEPPERS

239 CHICKEN BREAST WITH MUSTARD

241 SALMON WITH LEMON SAUCE AND DILL

SIDE DISH RECIPES

INTRODUCTION TO THE DISSOCIATED DIET

Origins and History Fundamental Principles

Origins and History The Dissociated Diet is a dietary regime that has gained popularity thanks to its distinctive approach to combining foods. Its roots can be traced to the early 20th century, with the work of Dr. William Howard Hay , an American physician. Hay developed what is known as the "food combination diet," which is based on the theory that the appropriate combination of foods can improve digestion and promote optimal health. Fundamental Principles The key principle of the Dissociated Diet is that certain food groups should not be consumed together in the same meal. This approach is based on the belief that the digestion of different types of foods requires different chemical conditions and digestion times.

Mixing proteins and carbohydrates, for example, could slow digestion and lead to weight gain and digestive problems. The basic principles of the diet include: 1. Separation of Food Groups: Protein foods and carbohydrate-rich foods should not be consumed in the same meal. Fruits and vegetables can be consumed freely, but they also have some combination rules. 2. Prioritize Simplicity: Meals should be simple, with few ingredients, to facilitate digestion and absorption of nutrients. 3. Time Intervals: It is recommended to wait a certain amount of time between meals to ensure that food is digested properly before introducing new foods into your system. The Dissociated Diet has been adopted by many people not only for weight loss, but also to improve overall well-being and digestion.

WHAT IS THE DISSOCIATED DIET

The Dissociated Diet is a diet based on a specific combination of foods that can be consumed together in one meal, while avoiding or limiting foods that are not compatible with each other. The basic idea is that some foods digest better when eaten separately, while others can be successfully combined. The main characteristics of the Dissociated Diet include: 1. Specific Combinations : Foods are grouped into categories, and an attempt is made to avoid consuming foods from different categories in the same meal. For example, meat and bread are often avoided in the same meal, while meat and vegetables can be eaten together. 2. Objective of Nutritional Balance: The diet seeks to achieve nutritional balance, allowing you to obtain a variety of essential nutrients from different food sources.

3. Portion Control : While food combinations are important, portion control remains an essential aspect of the diet. **4. Promoting Weight Loss:** The Dissociated Diet is often adopted by those who wish to lose weight, but it also focuses on maintaining a balanced and healthy diet. It is important to note that the Dissociated Diet is a controversial dietary approach, and there is no scientific consensus on its effectiveness. Some argue that specific food combinations do not have a solid scientific basis, while others claim to have achieved weight loss and well-being benefits. Before adopting any diet, it is advisable to consult a health professional or dietician to assess whether it is suitable for your needs and state of health. Choosing a diet should always be based on reliable information and a balanced nutritional plan.

HOW THE DISSOCIATED DIET WORKS

Division of Foods Allowed and Prohibited Food Combinations

The Dissociated Diet: Secrets, Combinations and How It Works

The Dissociated Diet, also known as the Hay Diet , is based on the idea that combining certain foods in the same meal can hinder digestion and absorption of nutrients.

Fundamental principles:

Separation of foods: Foods are divided into three categories: carbohydrates, proteins and starches. According to the diet, these groups should not be combined in the same meal.

Allowed Combinations: The diet allows some specific combinations, such as fruits and vegetables, vegetables and lean protein, or grains and fruit.

THE BENEFITS OF THE DISSOCIATED DIET

The Dissociated Diet has received attention from many people for its purported benefits, but it is important to note that scientific studies on the subject are limited, and the diet is a subject of debate among experts. However, some advocates of the Dissociated Diet claim that it has the following potential benefits: 1. Weight Loss : One of the main goals of the Dissociated Diet is weight loss. Separating food groups into separate meals can lead to a reduction in calorie intake, which could contribute to weight loss, especially when combined with adequate portion control. 2. Simplifying Food Choices: Dividing foods into separate groups simplifies food choices and can help people focus on healthier foods.

3. Improved Digestion: Some claim that the Dissociated Diet improves digestion because foods are digested more efficiently when consumed with other compatible foods. **4. Dietary Variation :** The diet promotes a variety of foods, encouraging the consumption of fruits, vegetables, lean meats and other healthful foods. Furthermore, the Dissociated Diet can be difficult to follow in the long term and could lead to a nutritional imbalance if not followed carefully. Before embarking on any diet, it is essential to consult a health professional or dietician to assess whether it is appropriate for your needs and state of health. Furthermore, it is always advisable to adopt a balanced approach to diet that promotes long-term health and is sustainable over time.

CONCLUSION FUTURE OF THE DISSOCIATED DIET

The Dissociated Diet 2025 represents an innovative and sustainable approach to improving health and well-being through the correct combination of foods. Through this book, we have explored the scientific basis, benefits, practical strategies and success stories of those who have already adopted this lifestyle. Conclusion Adopting the Dissociated Diet means embracing a positive and conscious change in the way you eat. The principles of this diet, based on the correct combination of foods, can lead to better digestion, increased energy and effective weight management. Furthermore, the attention to the simplicity and naturalness of the ingredients promotes a balanced diet rich in essential nutrients.

Remember, every small positive change in your diet can have a big impact on your long-term health.

The Future of the Dissociated Diet The future of the Dissociated Diet is promising. As scientific research in the field of nutrition advances, we can expect further insights into the benefits of food combinations and their impact on health. Furthermore, the integration of modern technologies, such as diet management apps and health monitoring tools, will make following this diet even easier and more accessible. We will continue to explore new recipes, personalized meal plans and practical tips for adapting the Dissociated Diet to individual needs.

RECIPES APPETIZERS

25

TOMATO AND CUCUMBER SALAD WITH OLIVE OIL

Preparation time: 15 minutes

Cooking times: None

Doses for 4 people

Ingredients:

4 ripe tomatoes

2 cucumbers

Extra virgin olive oil

Salt and black pepper

Preparation:

1. Cut the tomatoes and cucumbers into thin slices. 2. Arrange the tomato and cucumber slices on a serving plate. 3. Season with extra virgin olive oil, salt and black pepper to taste. 4. Serve immediately as a light and refreshing appetizer.

CAPRESE WITH LIGHT MOZZARELLA

Preparation time: 10 minutes

Cooking times: None

Doses for 4 people

Ingredients:

4 ripe tomatoes

200 g of light mozzarella

Fresh basil leaves

Extra virgin olive oil

Salt and black pepper

Preparation:

1. Cut the tomatoes and mozzarella into thin slices. 2. Alternate slices of tomato, mozzarella and basil leaves on a serving platter. 3. Season with extra virgin olive oil, salt and black pepper to taste. 4. Serve as a classic and tasty appetizer.

MELON AND RAW HAM SKEWERS

Preparation time: 15 minutes

Cooking times: None

Doses for 4 people

Ingredients:

1 ripe melon

100 g of raw ham

Wooden skewers

(to assemble)

Preparation:

1. Cut the melon into cubes or use a corer to make melon balls. 2. Wrap the melon pieces with slices of raw ham. 3. Thread the melon and ham morsels onto wooden skewers. 4. Serve as a fresh and tasty appetizer.

COURGETTE CARPACCIO WITH FRESH MINT

Preparation time: 20 minutes

Cooking times: None

Doses for 4 people

Ingredients:

2 courgettes

Lemon juice

Extra virgin olive oil

Fresh mint

Salt and black pepper

Preparation:

1. Cut the courgettes into thin slices. 2. Arrange the courgette slices on a serving plate. 3. Season with lemon juice, extra virgin olive oil, fresh mint, salt and black pepper to taste. 4. Serve as a light and refined appetizer.

GRILLED AUBERGINES WITH GARLIC AND CHILLI

Preparation time: 15 minutes

Cooking times: 10 minutes

Doses for 4 people

Ingredients:

2 aubergines

2 cloves of garlic

Fresh chili pepper or powder (to taste)

Extra virgin olive oil

Salt and black pepper

Preparation:

1. Cut the aubergines into thin slices. 2. Heat a grill and cook the aubergine slices until you get grill streaks on both sides. 3. In a pan, heat the olive oil with the garlic and chili pepper. Add the grilled aubergines and cook for a few minutes. 4. Season with salt and pepper to taste. Serve as a boldly flavored appetizer.

TUNA TARTARE WITH AVOCADO

Preparation time: 20 minutes

Cooking times: None

Doses for 4 people

Ingredients:

300 g of raw tuna

2 ripe avocados

Lemon juice

Red onion (optional)

Extra virgin olive oil

Salt and black pepper

Preparation:

1. Cut the tuna into small cubes. 2. Cut the avocados into cubes and sprinkle them with lemon juice. 3. Stir in the tuna, avocado, and red onion (if desired). 4. Season with olive oil, salt and pepper to taste. Serve as a sophisticated appetizer.

WHOLE WHOLE BRUSCHETTAS WITH TOMATOES AND BASIL

Preparation time: 15 minutes

Cooking times: 5 minutes

Doses for 4 people

Ingredients:

Whole grain bread

Cherry tomatoes

Fresh basil

Garlic

Extra virgin olive oil

Salt and black pepper

Preparation:

1. Cut the wholemeal bread into thick slices and grill them . 2. Cut the cherry tomatoes in half and chop the fresh basil. 3. Rub the bread slices with garlic. 4. Add the cherry tomatoes, basil, olive oil, salt and pepper. Serve as a crunchy appetizer.

SMOKED SALMON WITH LIGHT CREAM CHEESE

Preparation time: 10 minutes

Cooking times: None

Doses for 4 people

Ingredients:

200 g of smoked salmon

Light cream cheese

Fresh dill (optional)

Lemon

Wholemeal bread or wholemeal crackers

Preparation:

1. Arrange the smoked salmon slices on a serving plate. 2. Add a small amount of light cream cheese to each salmon slice. 3. Add fresh dill and a squeeze of lemon juice. 4. Serve with slices of wholemeal bread or wholemeal crackers . An elegant and tasty appetizer.

CHICKEN MEATBALLS WITH LEMON

Preparation time: 20 minutes

Cooking times: 15 minutes

Doses for 4 people

Ingredients:

500g minced chicken breast

Grated lemon (zest)

Chopped fresh parsley

Egg

Bread crumbs

Salt and black pepper

Preparation:

1. In a bowl, mix the minced chicken, lemon zest, parsley, egg, breadcrumbs, salt and pepper. 2. Form small meatballs with the dough. 3. Cook the meatballs in a pan with a drizzle of oil until golden brown on both sides. 4. Serve as a tasty appetizer.

SHRIMP AND AVOCADO SALAD

Preparation time: 15 minutes

Cooking times: 5 minutes

(for the shrimp, if necessary)

Doses for 4 people

Ingredients:

Boiled prawns

Ripe avocado

Lemon

Mixed salad

Extra virgin olive oil

Salt and black pepper

Preparation:

1. Cut the avocado into cubes and sprinkle it with lemon juice to avoid oxidation. 2. In a bowl, mix the mixed salad with the prawns. 3. Add the avocado and season with olive oil , salt and pepper to taste. 4. Serve as a fresh and healthy appetizer.

STEAMED VEGETABLES WITH YOGURT SAUCE

Preparation time: 15 minutes

Cooking times: 10 minutes

Doses for 4 people

Ingredients:

A variety of vegetables

(e.g. broccoli, carrots, courgettes)

Light yogurt

Herbs

(e.g. thyme, rosemary)

Salt and black pepper

Preparation:

1. Steam vegetables until tender but crunchy.
2. Make a yogurt sauce by mixing low-fat yogurt, chopped herbs, salt and pepper. 3. Serve steamed vegetables with yogurt sauce as a healthy appetizer.

AUBERGINE BALLS STUFFED WITH LIGHT CHEESE

Preparation time: 30 minutes

Cooking times: 20 minutes

Doses for 4 people

Ingredients:

Eggplant

Light cheese (e.g. cheese

light spreadable)

Dry tomatoes

Fresh basil

Salt and black pepper

Preparation:

1. Cut the aubergines into thin slices and grill them . 2. Prepare a cream by mixing the light cheese, chopped dried tomatoes, fresh basil, salt and pepper. 3. Lay out a slice of aubergine, put a small amount of cream cheese in the center and close into a ball. 4. Cook the aubergine balls in the oven until golden brown. 5. Serve as an elegant and tasty appetizer.

BOILED EGGS WITH LIGHT MAYONNAISE

Preparation time: 15 minutes

Cooking times: 10 minutes

Doses for 4 people

Ingredients:

Hard-boiled eggs

Light mayonnaise

Aromatic herbs (e.g. parsley)

Salt and black pepper

Preparation:

1. Peel the hard-boiled eggs and cut them in half. 2. Remove the egg yolks and mix with the light mayonnaise, chopped herbs, salt and pepper. 3. Fill the egg halves with the mixture. 4. Serve as a creamy and tasty appetizer.

ZUCCHINI FRITTERS

Preparation time: 20 minutes

Cooking times: 15 minutes

Doses for 4 people

Ingredients:

Zuchinis

Egg

wholemeal flour

Light grated cheese

Salt and black pepper

Preparation:

1. Grate the courgettes and squeeze them to remove excess water. 2. Mix the grated zucchini with eggs, wholemeal flour, light grated cheese, salt and pepper. 3. Cook the pancakes in a pan until golden brown on both sides. 4. Serve as a crunchy and healthy appetizer.

RAW HAM WITH FRESH FIGS

Preparation time: 10 minutes

Cooking times: None

Doses for 4 people

Ingredients:

Raw ham

Fresh figs

Balsamic vinegar (optional)

Preparation:

1. Wrap slices of raw ham around fresh figs.
2. You can serve with a touch of balsamic vinegar, if desired. 3. Serve as an elegant appetizer with a harmonious flavor.

STUFFED TOMATOES WITH TUNA AND ONION

Preparation time: 20 minutes

Cooking times: None

Doses for 4 people

Ingredients:

Ripe tomatoes

Canned tuna

Red onion

Black olives (optional)

Extra virgin olive oil

Salt and black pepper

Preparation:

1. Cut off the tops of the tomatoes and empty them . 2. Mix tuna, chopped red onion, black olives (if desired), olive oil, salt and pepper. 3. Fill the tomatoes with the mixture. 4. Serve as a fresh and tasty appetizer.

SALMON ROLL WITH SPREADABLE CHEESE

Preparation time: 20 minutes

Cooking times: None

Doses for 4 people

Ingredients:

Slices of smoked salmon

Light spreadable cheese

Aromatic herbs (e.g. dill)

Lemon Salt and black pepper

Preparation:

1. Lay out the smoked salmon slices on a work surface. 2. Spread the cream cheese on the salmon slices. 3. Add herbs, lemon juice, salt and pepper. 4. Roll up the salmon slices and cut them into small rolls . 5. Serve as a refined appetizer.

FENNEL SALAD WITH ORANGES

Preparation time: 15 minutes

Cooking times: None

Doses for 4 people

Ingredients:

Fennel

Oranges

Black olives (optional)

Extra virgin olive oil

Salt and black pepper

Preparation:

1. Finely slice the fennel and cut the oranges into slices. 2. Mix fennel, oranges, black olives (if desired), olive oil, salt and pepper. 3. Serve as a fresh and fragrant appetizer.

CARROT FLAN

55

Preparation time: 25 minutes

Cooking times: 30 minutes

Doses for 4 people

Ingredients:

Carrots

Egg

Light grated cheese

Light cream

Nutmeg

Salt and black pepper

Preparation:

1. Cook the carrots and blend them with eggs, light grated cheese, light cream, nutmeg, salt and pepper. 2. Pour the mixture into a baking tray and cook until golden. 3. Serve as a creamy and healthy appetizer.

MARINATED SALMON WITH CUCUMBERS AND LEMON

Preparation time: 30 minutes (marinade)

Cooking times: 10 minutes

Doses for 4 people

Ingredients:

Salmon fillets

Cucumbers

Lemon

Extra virgin olive oil

Fresh dill

Salt and black pepper

Preparation:

1. Prepare a marinade with olive oil, lemon juice, chopped fresh dill, salt and pepper. 2. Marinate the salmon fillets with the marinade for at least 30 minutes. 3. Cook the salmon in a pan until golden brown. 4. Serve with cucumber slices as a refreshing appetizer.

AVOCADO CREAM WITH WHOLE CROUTTONS

Preparation time: 15 minutes

Cooking times: None

Doses for 4 people

Ingredients:

Ripe avocado

Lemon

Wholemeal croutons

Extra virgin olive oil

Salt and black pepper

Preparation:

1. Blend the avocado with lemon juice, salt and pepper until smooth. 2. Spread the avocado cream on the wholemeal croutons. 3. Serve as a creamy and healthy appetizer.

MELON WITH

MINT SCENT

Preparation time: 10 minutes

Cooking times: None

Doses for 4 people

Ingredients:

Ripe melon

Fresh mint leaves

Lemon

Preparation:

1. Cut the melon into thin slices or make melon balls. 2. Add fresh mint leaves and a squeeze of lemon juice. 3. Serve as a refreshing appetizer.

TURKEY ROLLS WITH ARUGULA AND DRIED TOMATOES

Preparation time: 20 minutes

Cooking times: None

Doses for 4 people

Ingredients:

Thin turkey slices

Arugula

Dried Tomatoes in Oil

Light spreadable cheese

Salt and black pepper

Preparation:

1. Lay out turkey slices and spread light cream cheese on each slice. 2. Add arugula leaves and pieces of dried tomatoes. 3. Roll up the turkey slices and cut them into small rolls. 4. Serve as a tasty appetizer.

ASPARAGUS SALAD
WITH BOILED EGGS

Preparation time: 20 minutes

Cooking times: 10 minutes

Doses for 4 people

Ingredients:

Asparagus

Hard-boiled eggs

Mustard

Lemon

Extra virgin olive oil

Salt and black pepper

Preparation:

1. Steam the asparagus until tender but crunchy. 2. Make a sauce with mustard, lemon juice, olive oil, salt and pepper. 3. Mix the asparagus with the sliced hard-boiled eggs and the sauce. 4. Serve as a fresh and tasty appetizer.

BASKETS OF PARMESAN CHEESE WITH MIXED SALAD

Preparation time: 20 minutes

Cooking times: 10 minutes

Doses for 4 people

Ingredients:

Grated Parmesan cheese

Mixed salad

Cherry tomatoes

Black olives (optional)

Extra virgin olive oil

Balsamic vinegar

Salt and black pepper

Preparation:

1. Form small baskets with the grated parmesan and bake them in the oven until golden. 2. Prepare a mixed salad with mixed salad , cherry tomatoes, black olives, olive oil, balsamic vinegar, salt and pepper. 3. Fill the parmesan baskets with the salad. 4. Serve as a crunchy and tasty appetizer.

AUBERGINES FRITTERS WITH GREEK YOGURT

Preparation time: 30 minutes

Cooking times: 15 minutes

Doses for 4 people

Ingredients:

Aubergines

Egg

wholemeal flour

Light Greek yogurt

Fresh mint

Salt and black pepper

Preparation:

1. Cut the aubergines into thin slices and fry them in a pan until golden brown. 2. Make a batter with eggs, wholemeal flour, salt and pepper. 3. Dip the aubergine slices in the batter and fry until golden brown. 4. Prepare a sauce with light Greek yogurt, chopped fresh mint, salt and pepper. 5. Serve the aubergine fritters with the sauce as a crunchy and creamy appetizer.

PRAWNS IN LIGHT PINK SAUCE

Preparation time: 15 minutes

Cooking times: 5 minutes

Doses for 4 people

Ingredients:

Shrimp

Light Greek yogurt

Light ketchup

Worcestershire sauce

Lemon

Salt and black pepper

Preparation:

1. Cook the shrimp in a skillet until pink and tender. 2. Make a light pink sauce by mixing light Greek yogurt, light ketchup, Worcestershire sauce , lemon juice, salt and pepper. 3. Serve the prawns with the sauce as a fresh and tasty appetizer.

AVOCADO AND TOMATO TARTARE

Preparation time: 15 minutes

Cooking times: None

Doses for 4 people

Ingredients:

Ripe avocado

Ripe tomatoes

Red onion (optional)

Lime

Fresh coriander

Salt and black pepper

Preparation:

1. Cut the avocado and tomatoes into cubes.
2. Add chopped red onion (if desired), lime, chopped fresh cilantro, salt and pepper. 3. Gently mix the ingredients. 4. Serve the avocado and tomato tartare as a fresh and fragrant appetizer.

GRILLED VEGETABLES WITH BASIL PESTO

Preparation time: 30 minutes

Cooking times: 15 minutes

Doses for 4 people

Ingredients:

A variety of vegetables (e.g. courgettes, peppers, aubergines)

Basil pesto

Extra virgin olive oil

Salt and black pepper

Preparation:

1. Cut the vegetables into slices and grill them until tender but crunchy. 2. Toss the grilled vegetables with the basil pesto, olive oil, salt and pepper. 3. Serve as a Mediterranean-flavored appetizer.

STUFFED EGGS WITH TUNA AND OLIVES

Preparation time: 20 minutes

Cooking times: 10 minutes

Doses for 4 people

Ingredients:

Hard-boiled eggs

Canned tuna

Black olives

Light mayonnaise

Fresh parsley

Salt and black pepper

Preparation:

1. Peel the hard-boiled eggs and cut them in half. 2. Remove the egg yolks and mix with tuna, chopped black olives, light mayonnaise, chopped fresh parsley, salt and pepper. 3. Fill the egg halves with the mixture. 4. Serve as a creamy and tasty appetizer.

MUSHROOM CARPACCIO WITH ARUGULA AND PARMESAN FLAKES

75

Preparation time: 15 minutes

Cooking times: None

Doses for 4 people

Ingredients:

Fresh mushrooms (e.g. champignons)

Rocket

Grated Parmesan cheese

Lemon

Extra virgin olive oil

Salt and black pepper

Preparation:

1. Slice the mushrooms into thin slices. 2. Arrange the mushroom slices on a serving plate. 3. Add arugula leaves, parmesan flakes, lemon juice, olive oil, salt and pepper. 4. Serve as a fresh and refined appetizer.

COOKED HAM WITH MELON AND BASIL

Preparation time: 15 minutes

Cooking times: None

Doses for 4 people

Ingredients:

Slices of cooked ham

Ripe melon

Fresh basil leaves

Preparation:

1. Wrap slices of cooked ham around melon wedges. 2. Add fresh basil leaves. 3. Serve as a refreshing appetizer.

BRUSCHETTA WITH TOMATO, BASIL AND ONION

78

Preparation time: 15 minutes

Cooking times: None

Doses for 4 people

Ingredients:

Whole grain bread

Ripe tomatoes

Fresh basil leaves

Red onion

Extra virgin olive oil

Salt and black pepper

Preparation:

1. Toast the bread and cut it into slices. 2. Cut the tomatoes into cubes and the onion into thin slices. 3. Arrange the tomatoes, basil and onion on the bread slices. 4. Season with olive oil, salt and pepper. 5. Serve as a classic and tasty appetizer.

CHICKEN SALAD WITH CELERY AND APPLE

Preparation time: 20 minutes

Cooking times: 15 minutes

(for chicken, if necessary)

Doses for 4 people

Ingredients:

Chicken breast

Celery

Green apples

Nuts

Light Greek yogurt

Mustard

Lemon

Salt and black pepper

Preparation:

1. Cook the chicken breast and cut it into cubes. 2. Cut the celery into slices, the apples into cubes and the walnuts into small pieces. 3. Make a sauce with light Greek yogurt, mustard, lemon juice, salt and pepper. 4. Mix the ingredients and dressing to create a fresh, flavorful chicken salad.

CARPACCIO OF RADISH WITH WALNUTS AND LIGHT GORGONZOLA

Preparation time: 15 minutes

Cooking times: None

Doses for 4 people

Ingredients:

Radish

Nuts

Gorgonzola light

Extra virgin olive oil

Honey

Salt and black pepper

Preparation:

1. Cut the radicchio into thin slices. 2. Arrange the radicchio slices on a serving plate. 3. Add crumbled walnuts and pieces of light gorgonzola. 4. Season with olive oil, honey, salt and pepper. 5. Serve as a uniquely flavored appetizer.

GRILLED PRAWN SKEWERS

Preparation time: 20 minutes

Cooking times: 10 minutes

Doses for 4 people

Ingredients:

Fresh or frozen prawns

Lemon

Extra virgin olive oil

Garlic

Fresh parsley

Salt and black pepper

Preparation:

1. Marinate the shrimp with lemon juice, olive oil, minced garlic, fresh parsley, salt and pepper. 2. Thread shrimp onto skewers and grill until pink and tender. 3. Serve the prawn skewers as a succulent appetizer.

POACHED EGGS ON ROAST POTATOES

Preparation time: 30 minutes

Cooking times: 30 minutes

Doses for 4 people

Ingredients:

Eggs Potatoes

Fresh rosemary

Extra virgin olive oil

Salt and black pepper

Preparation:

1. Cut the potatoes into thin slices and roast them with rosemary, olive oil, salt and pepper until crispy. 2. Poach the eggs and serve on a bed of roasted potatoes. 3. Serve as a rustic appetizer.

GREEN BEANS WITH YOGURT SAUCE AND AROMATIC HERBS

Preparation time: 20 minutes

Cooking times: 10 minutes

Doses for 4 people

Ingredients:

Green beans

Light Greek yogurt

Herbs

(parsley, chives)

Lemon

Salt and black pepper

Preparation:

1. Steam the green beans until tender but crunchy. 2. Prepare a sauce with light Greek yogurt, chopped herbs, lemon juice, salt and pepper. 3. Season the green beans with the sauce. 4. Serve as a fresh and healthy appetizer.

GRATIN TOMATOES WITH WHOLEMEAL BREAD

Preparation time: 20 minutes

Cooking times: 15 minutes

Doses for 4 people

Ingredients:

Ripe tomatoes

Whole grain bread

Garlic

Origan

Grated Parmesan cheese

Salt and black pepper

Preparation:

1. Cut the tomatoes in half and remove the seeds. 2. Chop the wholemeal bread, garlic, oregano, grated Parmesan, salt and pepper in a blender. 3. Fill the tomatoes with the mixture and grill them in the oven until golden. 4. Serve as a crunchy and tasty appetizer.

COURGETTE ROLLS FILLED WITH LIGHT RICOTTA

Preparation time: 30 minutes

Cooking times: 15 minutes

Doses for 4 people

Ingredients:

Zuchinis

Light ricotta

Nutmeg

Light grated cheese

Salt and black pepper

Preparation:

1. Cut the courgettes into thin slices and cook them briefly in boiling water. 2. Prepare a filling with light ricotta, nutmeg, light grated cheese, salt and pepper. 3. Fill the courgette slices with the filling and roll them up . 4. Cook the rolls until golden brown. 5. Serve as a creamy and healthy appetizer.

RECIPES
FIRST DISHES

COURGETTE SPAGHETTI WITH BASIL PESTO

preparation time: 20 minutes

cooking times: 10 minutes

doses for 4 people

ingredients:

Courgettes (500 g)

Fresh basil (1 bunch)

Almonds or pine nuts (50 g)

Light grated cheese (30 g)

Garlic (1 clove)

Extra virgin olive oil (60 ml)

Salt and black pepper

Preparation: 1.

Use a spiralizer to create zucchini noodles. 2. Make a pesto by blending fresh basil, almonds or pine nuts, light grated cheese, garlic, olive oil, salt and pepper. 3. Season the courgette spaghetti with the basil pesto. 4. Serve as a fresh and light dish.

WHOLE WHOLE RISOTTO WITH PORCINI MUSHROOMS

preparation time: 10 minutes

cooking times: 3040 minutes

doses for 4 people

ingredients:

Brown rice (350 g)

Fresh or dried porcini mushrooms (200 g)

Onion (1)

Vegetable broth (1.2 l)

Dry white wine (120 ml)

Light butter (30 g)

Light grated cheese (30 g)

Salt and black pepper

Preparation:

1. Brown the onion in a little light butter. 2. Add the brown rice and toast it lightly. 3. Add the porcini mushrooms and blend with the dry white wine. 4. Add the vegetable broth gradually and cook the risotto until cooked. 5. Cream with light butter and light grated cheese. 6. Complete with chopped fresh parsley, salt and pepper. 7. Serve as a main course full of flavour.

WHOLEWHEAT PENNE WITH TOMATOES AND OLIVES

preparation time: 15 minutes

cooking times: 15 minutes

doses for 4 people

ingredients:

Wholemeal penne (360 g)

Cherry tomatoes (250 g)

Black olives (50 g)

Garlic (2 cloves)

Extra virgin olive oil (60 ml)

Fresh basil

Salt and black pepper

Preparation:

1. Cook the wholemeal penne in salted water until al dente. 2. In a pan, sauté garlic in olive oil, then add cherry tomatoes and olives. 3. Cook for a few minutes, then add the cooked penne. 4. Season with fresh basil, salt and pepper. 5. Serve as a simple but tasty main course.

LENTIL SOUP WITH CELERY AND CARROTS

preparation time: 15 minutes

cooking times: 3040 minutes

doses for 4 people

ingredients:

Dried lentils (250 g)

Celery (2 stalks)

Carrots (2)

Onion (1)

Vegetable broth (1.5 l)

Fresh rosemary

Salt and black pepper

Preparation:

1. Brown onion, celery and carrots in a pan with a little olive oil. 2. Add dried lentils and vegetable broth. 3. Cook until lentils are tender. 4. Add fresh rosemary, salt and pepper. 5. Serve as a warm, nutritious soup.

CUCUMBER NOODLES WITH LEMON SAUCE

preparation time: 20 minutes

cooking times: None

doses for 4 people

ingredients:

Cucumbers (4)

Lemon (2)

Light Greek yogurt (200 g)

Fresh mint (10 leaves)

Salt and black pepper

Preparation:

1. Use a spiralizer to make cucumber noodles. 2. Prepare a sauce with lemon juice, light Greek yogurt, chopped fresh mint, salt and pepper. 3. Season the cucumber noodles with the lemon sauce. 4. Serve as a fresh and light dish.

LIGHT ZUCCHINI AND RICOTTA LASAGNE

preparation time: 30 minutes

cooking times: 30/40 minutes

doses for 4 people

ingredients:

Courgettes (4)

Light ricotta (300 g)

Tomato (400 g)

Garlic (2 cloves)

Light grated cheese (50 g)

Fresh basil

Salt and black pepper

Preparation:

1. Cut the courgettes into thin slices and grill them until tender but crunchy. 2. Prepare a layer of grilled courgettes, light ricotta, tomato, garlic, light grated cheese, fresh basil, salt and pepper. 3. Repeat the layers to create the lasagna. 4. Bake in the oven until golden brown. 5. Serve as a light main course.

BASMATI RICE WITH GRILLED VEGETABLES

preparation time: 20 minutes

cooking times: 15 minutes

doses for 4 people

ingredients:

Basmati rice (350 g)

Mixed vegetables (e.g. peppers,

courgettes, aubergines) (400 g)

Extra virgin olive oil (60 ml)

Aromatic herbs to taste

(e.g. thyme, rosemary)

Salt and black pepper

Preparation:

1. Cook the basmati rice as directed on the package. 2. Grill mixed vegetables with olive oil, herbs, salt and pepper. 3. Mix the cooked rice with the grilled vegetables. 4. Serve as a healthy and tasty main course.

TOMATO SOUP

WITH FRESH BASIL

preparation time: 15 minutes

cooking times: 30 minutes

doses for 4 people

ingredients:

Ripe tomatoes (800 g)

Onion (1)

Garlic (2 cloves)

Vegetable broth (1.2 l)

Fresh basil

Salt and black pepper

Preparation:

1. Brown the onion and garlic in a pan with a little olive oil. 2. Add diced ripe tomatoes and cook until soft. 3. Add vegetable broth and fresh basil. 4. Blend the soup until it becomes smooth. 5. Serve as a hot, fragrant soup.

CARROT SPAGHETTI WITH AVOCADO SAUCE

Preparation time: 15 minutes

Cooking times: 1012 minutes

Doses for 4 people

Ingredients:

Carrot spaghetti (400 g)

Avocados (2)

Lemon (1)

Fresh basil

Extra virgin olive oil (60 ml)

Salt and black pepper

Preparation:

1. Cook the carrot spaghetti in boiling water until al dente. 2. Make a sauce by blending avocado, lemon juice, fresh basil, olive oil, salt and pepper. 3. Pour the sauce over the carrot spaghetti. 4. Serve as a fresh and colorful main course.

STEAMED RAVIOLI WITH SPINACH AND RICOTTA

Preparation time: 20 minutes

Cooking times: 810 minutes

Doses for 4 people

Ingredients:

Ravioli (400 g)

Fresh spinach (200 g)

Ricotta (200 g)

Butter (60 g)

Fresh sage

Salt and black pepper

Preparation:

1. Cook the ravioli in boiling water until al dente. 2. In a skillet, sauté fresh spinach in butter until wilted. 3. Add the ricotta and mix until you get a creamy sauce. 4. Serve the steamed ravioli with the spinach and ricotta sauce. 5. Complete with sage leaves, salt and pepper.

RISOTTO WITH SAFFRON AND ASPARAGUS

Preparation time: 20 minutes

Cooking times: 1820 minutes

Doses for 4 people

Ingredients:

Arborio rice (320 g)

Saffron (1 sachet)

Asparagus (200 g)

Onion (1)

Dry white wine (120 ml)

Vegetable broth (1 litre)

Butter (60 g)

Parmesan cheese

grated (60 g)

Salt and black pepper

Preparation:

1. In a saucepan, sauté the chopped onion in butter until translucent. 2. Add the Arborio rice and toast it for a minute. 3. Pour in the dry white wine and cook until it has evaporated. 4. Add saffron and begin gradually adding the hot vegetable broth, stirring constantly. 5. Halfway through cooking, add the chopped asparagus. 6. Continue cooking until the rice is al dente and the risotto is creamy. 7. Top with grated Parmesan cheese, salt and pepper. 8. Serve as a delicate main course.

WHOLE FARFALLE WITH AUBERGINES AND TOMATOES

Preparation time: 15 minutes

Cooking times: 1520 minutes

Doses for 4 people

Ingredients:

Wholemeal farfalle (400 g)

Eggplants (2)

Cherry tomatoes (250 g)

Garlic (2 cloves)

Fresh basil

Extra virgin olive oil (60 ml)

Salt and black pepper

Preparation:

1. Cook whole farfalle in boiling water until al dente. 2. In a skillet, sauté minced garlic with diced eggplant in olive oil until golden . 3. Add cherry tomatoes halfway through cooking and cook until soft. 4. Top with fresh basil, salt and pepper. 5. Serve as a colorful and tasty main course.

MINESTRONE WITH LEGUMES AND MIXED VEGETABLES

Preparation time: 20 minutes

Cooking times: 40 minutes

Doses for 4 people

Ingredients:

Dried mixed legumes (200 g)

Mixed vegetables (e.g. courgettes, carrots, celery) (400 g)

Onion (1)

Vegetable broth (1.2 l)

Ripe tomatoes (400 g)

Extra virgin olive oil (60 ml)

Fresh parsley

Salt and black pepper

Preparation:

1. Soak the dried legumes in cold water for a few hours. 2. In a pan, brown the onion with olive oil. 3. Add the diced mixed vegetables and cook for a few minutes. 4. Add the drained legumes, the diced ripe tomatoes and the vegetable broth. 5. Cook until the legumes are tender. 6. Complete with chopped fresh parsley, salt and pepper. 7. Serve as a nutritious soup.

PENNE ALLA NORMA WITH AUBERGINES AND TOMATO

Preparation time: 20 minutes

Cooking times: 20 minutes

Doses for 4 people

Ingredients:

Wholemeal penne (360 g)

Eggplant Tomato (400 g)

Garlic (2 cloves)

Extra virgin olive oil (60 ml)

Fresh basil

Salt and black pepper

Preparation:

1. Cut the aubergines into cubes and cook them in a pan with olive oil until golden brown. 2. In a separate pan, sauté garlic in olive oil and add diced tomato. 3. Cook until you get a thick sauce. 4. Cook the wholemeal penne in salted water until al dente. 5. Mix the penne with the tomato sauce, aubergines and fresh basil. 6. Serve as a delicious main course.

WILD RICE WITH MUSHROOMS AND PARSLEY

Preparation time: 15 minutes

Cooking times: 45 minutes

Doses for 4 people

Ingredients:

Wild rice (250 g)

Mixed mushrooms

(e.g. porcini mushrooms, mushrooms) (300 g)

Onion (1)

Vegetable broth (1.2 l)

Fresh parsley

Extra virgin olive oil (60 ml)

Salt and black pepper

Preparation:

1. Brown the onion in olive oil until golden brown. 2. Add the sliced mushrooms and cook until golden. 3. Add the wild rice and toast it lightly. 4. Add the vegetable broth and cook until the rice is tender. 5. Complete with chopped fresh parsley, salt and pepper. 6. Serve as a rustic main course.

PEA SOUP WITH FRESH MINT

Preparation time: 15 minutes

Cooking times: 30 minutes

Doses for 4 people

Ingredients:

Peas (400 g)

Onion (1)

Vegetable broth (1.2 l)

Fresh mint (1 bunch)

Extra virgin olive oil (60 ml)

Salt and black pepper

Preparation:

1. In a saucepan, heat the olive oil and add the chopped onion. Sauté the onion over medium heat until translucent. 2. Add the peas and diced potatoes to the pot. Mix well and cook for a few minutes. 3. Pour the vegetable broth into the pot, cover with a lid and cook over medium heat for about 1520 minutes, or until the potatoes and peas are tender. 4. Use an immersion blender to blend the soup until smooth. 5. Add chopped fresh mint to the soup. Mix well. 6. Taste and add salt and black pepper to taste. 7. Serve the soup hot, garnished with a few fresh mint leaves on top. This pea soup with fresh mint is light and refreshing, perfect for a light dinner or appetizer.

PUMPKIN FETTUCCINE WITH PARSLEY PESTO

Preparation time: 20 minutes

Cooking times: 15 minutes

Doses for 4 people 5.

Ingredients:

Pumpkin fettuccine (340 g)

Pumpkin (200 g) Walnuts (50 g)

Fresh parsley

Extra virgin olive oil (60 ml)

Light grated cheese (30 g)

Salt and black pepper

Preparation:

1. Cook the pumpkin fettuccine in salted water until al dente. 2. Cook the diced pumpkin in a pan with olive oil. 3. Make a pesto by blending walnuts, fresh parsley, olive oil, light grated cheese, salt and pepper. 4. Season the pumpkin fettuccine with the cooked pumpkin and parsley pesto. 5. Serve as a delicious main course.

RICOTTA AND SPINACH RAVIOLI WITH TOMATO SAUCE

Preparation time: 20 minutes

Cooking times: 15 minutes

Doses for 4 people

Ingredients:

Ravioli stuffed with ricotta and spinach

Tomato (400 g)

Garlic (2 cloves)

Extra virgin olive oil (60 ml)

Fresh basil

Salt and black pepper

Preparation:

1. Cook the stuffed ravioli in boiling water until cooked. 2. In a pan, brown the garlic in olive oil. 3. Add diced tomato and cook until you get a thick sauce. 4. Drain the ravioli and toss them in the pan with the tomato sauce. 5. Top with fresh basil, salt and pepper. 6. Serve as a delicious main course.

CUCUMBER SPAGHETTI WITH PRAWNS AND AVOCADO

Preparation time: 20 minutes

Cooking times: 10 minutes

Doses for 4 people

Ingredients:

Cucumbers (4)

Prawns (200 g)

Ripe avocado

Lemon

Extra virgin olive oil (60 ml)

Salt and black pepper

Preparation:

1. Use a spiralizer to create cucumber noodles. 2. Cook the prawns in a pan with olive oil and lemon. 3. Make a sauce with ripe avocado, lemon juice, olive oil, salt and pepper. 4. Season the cucumber noodles with the shrimp and avocado sauce. 5. Serve as a fresh and light dish.

LEMON RISOTTO WITH ASPARAGUS

Preparation time: 15 minutes

Cooking times: 3040 minutes

Doses for 4 people

Ingredients:

Arborio rice (350 g)

Asparagus

Lemon

Vegetable broth (1.2 l)

Light butter (30 g)

Light grated cheese (30 g)

Salt and black pepper

Preparation:

1. Brown the asparagus in a pan with light butter. 2. Add the Arborio rice and toast it lightly. 3. Blend with lemon juice and zest and cook the risotto, gradually adding the vegetable broth. 4. Cream with light butter and light grated cheese. 5. Complete with salt and pepper. 6. Serve as a light and aromatic main course.

PEARL BARLEY WITH TOMATOES AND ARUGULA

Preparation time: 15 minutes

Cooking times: 2025 minutes

Doses for 4 people

Ingredients:

Pearl barley (330 g)

Cherry tomatoes (250 g)

Arugula

Garlic (2 cloves)

Extra virgin olive oil (60 ml)

Light grated cheese (30 g)

Salt and black pepper

Preparation:

1. Brown the garlic in olive oil in a pan. 2. Add the pearl barley and toast lightly. 3. Add halved cherry tomatoes and cook until orzo is tender. 4. Season with fresh arugula, light grated cheese, salt and pepper. 5. Serve as a tasty main course.

WHOLE WHOLE TAGLIATELLE WITH TOMATO SAUCE

Preparation time: 15 minutes

Cooking times: 1520 minutes

Doses for 4 people

Ingredients:

Wholemeal tagliatelle (360 g)

Tomato (400 g)

Garlic (2 cloves)

Fresh basil

Extra virgin olive oil (60 ml)

Salt and black pepper

Preparation:

1. Brown the garlic in olive oil in a pan. 2. Add diced tomatoes and cook until you get a thick sauce. 3. Cook the wholemeal tagliatelle in salted water until al dente. 4. Drain them and sauté them in the pan with the tomato sauce. 5. Top with fresh basil, salt and pepper. 6. Serve as a classic main course.

CAULIFLOWER SOUP WITH TOASTED NUTS

Preparation time: 15 minutes

Cooking times: 3040 minutes

Doses for 4 people

Ingredients:

Cauliflower (1)

Onion (1)

Walnuts (50 g)

Vegetable broth (1.2 l)

Light cream (120 ml)

Extra virgin olive oil (60 ml)

Salt and black pepper

Preparation:

1. Brown the onion in olive oil in a pan. 2. Add chopped cauliflower and cook until soft. 3. Blend the soup with vegetable broth and light cream. 4. Toast the walnuts in a pan without oil. 5. Serve the soup with toasted walnuts, salt and pepper. 6. Serve as a creamy, crunchy soup.

PAPPARDELLE WITH

LEAN MEAT SAUCE

Preparation time: 20 minutes

Cooking times: 60 minutes

Doses for 4 people

Ingredients:

300 g pappardelle (or pasta of your choice)

250g lean minced meat (chicken,

turkey or lean beef)

1 onion, finely chopped

2 cloves garlic, minced

1 carrot, chopped

1 stalk celery, chopped

400 g of peeled tomatoes

1 glass of red wine

Extra virgin olive oil

Salt and black pepper to taste

Fresh basil leaves for garnish

Grated cheese (Parmesan

or Pecorino) to serve

Preparation

1. In a large skillet, heat some olive oil over medium heat. Add the chopped onion, garlic, carrot and celery and fry until soft and golden. 2. Add the ground beef and cook until browned, breaking it up with a wooden spoon so it is evenly cooked. 3. Pour the red wine into the pan and let the alcohol evaporate. 4. Add the peeled tomatoes and break them up with a fork. Mix well and leave to cook over medium heat for approximately 2030 minutes, or until the ragù has thickened.

Add salt and pepper to taste. 5. Meanwhile, cook the pappardelle in boiling salted water following the instructions on the package. 6. Drain the pappardelle al dente and transfer them to the pan with the ragù. Mix well to blend the flavors. 7. Serve the pappardelle with the lean meat sauce, garnished with fresh basil leaves and a generous sprinkling of grated cheese. This recipe will give you a rich and flavorful dish, perfect for gourmets.

POTATO GNOCCHI WITH ARUGULA PESTO

Preparation time: 20 minutes

Cooking times: 5 minutes

Doses for 4 people

Ingredients:

Potato gnocchi (400 g)

Arugula

Walnuts (50 g)

Light grated cheese (30 g)

Extra virgin olive oil (60 ml)

Garlic (2 cloves)

Salt and black pepper

Preparation:

1. Cook the gnocchi in boiling water until they rise to the surface. 2. Make a pesto by blending arugula, walnuts, garlic, olive oil, light grated cheese, salt and pepper. 3. Season the gnocchi with the Arugula pesto. 4. Serve as a main course full of flavour.

BASMATI RICE WITH CURRY VEGETABLES

Preparation time: 15 minutes

Cooking times: 20 minutes

Doses for 4 people

Ingredients:

Basmati rice (350 g)

Mixed vegetables (e.g. peppers, courgettes, carrots) (400 g)

Onion (1)

Curry powder

Extra virgin olive oil (60 ml)

Salt and black pepper

Preparation:

1. Brown the onion in olive oil in a pan. 2. Add the diced mixed vegetables and cook for a few minutes. 3. Add curry powder and mix well. 4. Cook the basmati rice according to the instructions on the package. 5. Mix the rice with the curry vegetables, salt and pepper. 6. Serve as a fragrant main course.

BROCCOLI SOUP WITH LIGHT CHEESE

Preparation time: 15 minutes

Cooking times: 3040 minutes

Doses for 4 people

Ingredients:

Broccoli (1)

Onion (1)

Light cheese (150 g)

Vegetable broth (1.2 l)

Extra virgin olive oil (60 ml)

Salt and black pepper

Preparation:

1. Brown the onion in olive oil in a pan. 2. Add the chopped broccoli and cook until soft. 3. Blend the soup with light cheese and vegetable broth. 4. Bring to the boil and cook for a few minutes. 5. Serve as a light, creamy soup.

WHOLE WHOLE PENNE WITH TURNIP AND ANCHOVIES

Preparation time: 15 minutes

Cooking times: 15 minutes

Doses for 4 people

Ingredients:

Wholemeal penne (320 g)

Turnip greens

Anchovies in oil (50 g)

Garlic (2 cloves)

Extra virgin olive oil (60 ml)

Chili pepper (to taste)

Salt and black pepper

Preparation:

1. Cook the wholemeal penne in salted water until al dente. 2. In a pan, brown the garlic and chili pepper in olive oil. 3. Add the turnip greens and cook for a few minutes. 4. Add the anchovies in oil and cook until soft. 5. Drain the penne and toss them in the pan with the sauce. 6. Serve as a tasty main course.

SEAFOOD RISOTTO

Preparation time: 20 minutes

Cooking times: 2530 minutes

Doses for 4 people

Ingredients:

Arborio rice (320 g)

Mixed seafood (e.g. prawns, mussels, calamari) (400 g)

Garlic (2 cloves)

Dry white wine (120 ml)

Fish broth (1.2 l)

Extra virgin olive oil (60 ml)

Fresh parsley

Salt and black pepper

Preparation:

1. In a saucepan, sauté the garlic in olive oil.
2. Add the Arborio rice and toast it lightly. 3.
Add the dry white wine and cook until
evaporated. 4. Add the mixed seafood and
start cooking the risotto, gradually adding
the fish stock. 5. Stir in chopped fresh
parsley, salt and pepper. 6. Serve as a main
course full of flavour.

COURGETTE LINGUINE WITH TOMATO AND OLIVE SAUCE

Preparation time: 20 minutes

Cooking times: 1520 minutes

Doses for 4 people

Ingredients:

Courgette linguine (360 g)

Tomato (400 g)

Pitted black olives (50 g)

Garlic (2 cloves)

Extra virgin olive oil (60 ml)

Fresh basil

Salt and black pepper

Preparation:

1. In a pan, brown the garlic in olive oil. 2. Add diced tomatoes and pitted black olives, cook until you get a thick sauce. 3. Cook the courgette linguine in salted water until al dente. 4. Drain them and sauté them in the pan with the tomato and olive sauce. 5. Top with fresh basil, salt and pepper. 6. Serve as a light and tasty main course.

CHICKEN LASAGNA WITH SPINACH

Preparation time: 30 minutes

Cooking times: 4045 minutes

Doses for 4 people

Ingredients:

Lasagna sheets (320 g)

Chicken breast (400 g)

Fresh spinach

Light grated cheese (150 g)

Light béchamel (200 ml)

Light butter (30 g)

Salt and black pepper

Preparation:

1. Cook the chicken breast and cut it into pieces. 2. Prepare a layer of lasagna sheets, chicken breast, spinach, light béchamel sauce, light grated cheese, salt and pepper. 3. Continue alternating layers until you run out of ingredients. 4. Cook in a preheated oven at 180°C for 4045 minutes, or until the surface is golden. 5. Serve as a gratin main course.

BLACK RICE WITH ROASTED PEPPERS

Preparation time: 15 minutes

Cooking times: 4550 minutes

Doses for 4 people

Ingredients:

Black rice (320 g)

Red and yellow peppers (2)

Onion (1)

Vegetable broth (1.2 l)

Extra virgin olive oil (60 ml)

Sweet paprika

Salt and black pepper

Preparation:

1. Cook black rice according to package instructions. 2. Roast the peppers in the oven until the skin is black, then peel and cut into strips. 3. In a pan, brown the onion in olive oil. 4. Add the roasted peppers, black rice, sweet paprika, salt and pepper. 5. Cook for a few minutes. 6. Serve as a colorful main course.

BLACK BEAN SOUP WITH CORIANDER

Preparation time: 20 minutes

Cooking times: 11.5 hours

Doses for 4 people

Ingredients:

Dried black beans (360 g)

Onion (1)

Fresh coriander

Vegetable broth (1.2 l)

Extra virgin olive oil (60 ml)

Garlic (2 cloves)

Salt and black pepper

Preparation:

1. Soak dried black beans for at least 6 hours. 2. In a pan, brown the onion in olive oil. 3. Add chopped garlic and coriander and cook for a few minutes. 4. Add the soaked black beans and vegetable broth. 5. Simmer until the beans are soft. 6. Serve the soup with fresh coriander, salt and pepper. 7. Serve as a tasty main course.

WHOLE WHOLE FUSILLI WITH AUBERGINES AND DRIED TOMATOES

Preparation time: 20 minutes

Cooking times: 2025 minutes

Doses for 4 people

Ingredients:

Wholemeal fusilli (350 g)

Eggplant (2)

Dried tomatoes (50 g)

Garlic (2 cloves)

Extra virgin olive oil (60 ml)

Fresh basil

Salt and black pepper

Preparation:

1. Cut the aubergines into cubes and cook them in a pan with olive oil until tender. 2. Add chopped garlic and dried tomatoes cut into strips, cook for a few minutes. 3. Cook the wholemeal fusilli in salted water until al dente. 4. Drain them and sauté them in the pan with the aubergines and dried tomatoes. 5. Top with fresh basil, salt and pepper. 6. Serve as a tasty main course.

SHIITAKE MUSHROOM RISOTTO

Preparation time: 20 minutes

Cooking times: 2025 minutes

Doses for 4 people

Ingredients:

Arborio rice (350 g)

shiitake mushrooms (250 g)

Onion (1)

Dry white wine (120 ml)

Vegetable broth (1.2 l)

Light butter (30 g)

Salt and black pepper

Preparation:

1. In a saucepan, brown the onion in light butter. 2. Add the sliced shiitake mushrooms and cook until golden. 3. Add the Arborio rice and toast it lightly. 4. Add the dry white wine and cook until evaporated. 5. Gradually add the vegetable broth as you cook the risotto. 6. Stir in light butter, salt and pepper. 7. Serve as a main course full of flavour.

CARROT TAGLIATELLE WITH BASIL PESTO

Preparation time: 15 minutes

Cooking times: 1012 minutes

Doses for 4 people

Ingredients:

Carrot tagliatelle (380 g)

Fresh basil

Walnuts (50 g)

Light grated parmesan (30 g)

Extra virgin olive oil (60 ml)

Garlic (1 clove)

Salt and black pepper

Preparation:

1. Cook the carrot tagliatelle in salted water until al dente. 2. Make a pesto by blending basil, walnuts, garlic, olive oil, light grated Parmesan, salt and pepper. 3. Season the carrot tagliatelle with the basil pesto. 4. Serve as a light and colorful main course.

PUMPKIN GNOCCHI WITH BUTTER AND SAGE

Preparation time: 30 minutes

Cooking times: 1015 minutes

Doses for 4 people

Ingredients:

Pumpkin gnocchi (400 g)

Pumpkin (300 g)

Light butter (60 g)

Fresh sage

Salt and black pepper

Preparation:

1. Cook the pumpkin and mash it to obtain the puree. 2. In a pan, melt light butter and add fresh sage leaves. 3. Cook the pumpkin gnocchi in salted water until they rise to the surface. 4. Drain the gnocchi and season them with the pumpkin puree, butter and sage. 5. Complete with salt and pepper. 6. Serve as a fragrant main course.

BASMATI RICE WITH VEGETABLE CURRY

Preparation time: 20 minutes

Cooking times: 2025 minutes

Doses for 4 people

Ingredients:

Basmati rice (340 g)

Mixed vegetables (e.g. peppers, courgettes, carrots) (400 g)

Onion (1)

Curry powder

Extra virgin olive oil (60 ml)

Salt and black pepper

Preparation:

1. Brown the onion in olive oil in a pan. 2. Add the diced mixed vegetables and cook for a few minutes. 3. Add curry powder and mix well. 4. Cook the basmati rice according to the instructions on the package. 5. Mix the rice with the curry vegetables, salt and pepper. 6. Serve as a fragrant main course.

QUINOA MINESTRONE WITH SEASONAL VEGETABLES

Preparation time: 20 minutes

Cooking times: 3035 minutes

Doses for 4 people

Ingredients:

Quinoa (200g)

Seasonal vegetables (e.g. courgettes ,

green beans, carrots) (400 g)

Onion (1)

Vegetable broth (1.2 l)

Extra virgin olive oil (60 ml)

Fresh thyme

Salt and black pepper

Preparation:

1. In a pan, brown the onion in olive oil. 2. Add the chopped seasonal vegetables and cook for a few minutes. 3. Add the quinoa and vegetable broth. 4. Simmer until the quinoa is cooked and the vegetables are tender. 5. Serve with fresh thyme leaves, salt and pepper. 6. Serve as a nutritious minestrone soup.

WHOLE BUTTERFLIES WITH COURGETTE AND MINT CREAM

Preparation time: 20 minutes

Cooking times: 1520 minutes

Doses for 4 people

Ingredients:

Wholemeal Butterflies (320 g)

Courgettes (2)

Fresh mint

Light cream (200 ml)

Extra virgin olive oil (60 ml)

Garlic (2 cloves)

Salt and black pepper

Preparation:

1. Brown the garlic in olive oil in a pan. 2. Add sliced courgettes and cook until tender. 3. Add fresh mint and light cream, cook for a few minutes. 4. Cook the whole farfalle in salted water until al dente. 5. Drain them and season them with the courgette and mint cream. 6. Complete with salt and pepper. 7. Serve as a light and fragrant main course.

RECIPES
SECOND DISHES

GRILLED CHICKEN BREAST WITH LEMON SAUCE

Preparation time: 15 minutes

Cooking times: 1520 minutes

Doses for 4 people

Ingredients:

Chicken breast (4 pieces)

Lemon (2)

Extra virgin olive oil (60 ml)

Garlic (2 cloves)

Fresh parsley

Salt and black pepper

Preparation:

1. Marinate the chicken breast with lemon juice, minced garlic, olive oil, fresh parsley, salt and pepper. 2. Heat the grill and cook the chicken breast until browned and cooked through. 3. Make a lemon sauce with lemon juice, olive oil, minced garlic, fresh parsley, salt and pepper. 4. Serve the chicken breast with the lemon sauce. 5. Serve as a light and tasty main course.

STEAMED SALMON WITH YOGURT SAUCE

Preparation time: 20 minutes

Cooking times: 1520 minutes

Doses for 4 people

Ingredients:

4 salmon fillets (150 g each)

Low-fat yogurt (200 g)

Lemon (1)

Fresh dill

Salt and black pepper

Preparation:

1. Marinate the salmon with lemon juice, salt, pepper and fresh dill. 2. Steam the salmon until well cooked. 3. Make a yogurt sauce with low-fat yogurt, lemon juice, fresh dill, salt and pepper. 4. Serve the salmon with the yogurt sauce. 5. Serve as a light, protein-rich main course.

TURKEY CUTLET WITH A SIDE OF STEAMED VEGETABLES

Preparation time: 20 minutes

Cooking times: 1520 minutes

Doses for 4 people

Ingredients:

4 turkey cutlets (150 g each)

Mixed vegetables for the side dish

(e.g. broccoli, carrots, green beans)

Extra virgin olive oil (60 ml)

Salt and black pepper

Preparation:

1. Cook turkey cutlets in a pan with olive oil until golden brown and cooked through. 2. Steam the mixed vegetables until tender but crunchy. 3. Complete the side dish with salt and pepper. 4. Serve the turkey cutlets with a side of steamed vegetables. 5. Serve as a light and balanced main course.

LEAN BEEF STEAK WITH MUSHROOMS

Preparation time: 15 minutes

Cooking times: 1015 minutes

Doses for 4 people

Ingredients:

4 beef steaks

lean (150 g. each)

Mushrooms (200 g)

Onion (1)

Garlic (2 cloves)

Fresh rosemary

Salt and black pepper

Preparation:

1. Brown the onion and garlic in a pan with olive oil. 2. Add the beef steaks and cook until desired doneness. 3. In a separate pan, cook the mushrooms with fresh rosemary. 4. Complete with salt and pepper. 5. Serve the beef steaks with mushrooms as a side dish. 6. Serve as a protein-rich main course.

COD FILLET WITH AROMATIC HERBS CRUST

Preparation time: 15 minutes

Cooking times: 15/20 minutes

Doses for 4 people

Ingredients:

Cod fillets (4 pieces

200 g. each)

Mixed aromatic herbs

(e.g. parsley ,

basil, thyme)

Wholemeal breadcrumbs (60 g)

Lemon (1)

Extra virgin olive oil (60 ml)

Salt and black pepper

Preparation:

1. Mix wholemeal breadcrumbs with chopped herbs, grated lemon zest, olive oil, salt and pepper. 2. Press the herb crust onto the cod fillets. 3. Cook the cod fillets in the oven until the crust is golden and the fish is cooked. 4. Serve with lemon wedges. 5. Serve as a light and tasty main course.

CHICKEN WITH ALMONDS
WITH BROCCOLI

Preparation time: 20 minutes

Cooking times: 15/20 minutes

Doses for 4 people

Ingredients:

Chicken breast (4 pieces 150 g each)

Broccoli (400 g)

Almonds (50 g)

Garlic (2 cloves)

Extra virgin olive oil (60 ml)

Fresh ginger

Salt and black pepper

Preparation:

1. Cut the chicken breast into strips and cook in a pan with olive oil, chopped garlic, grated fresh ginger, salt and pepper. 2. In a separate pan, steam the broccoli until tender. 3. Toast the almonds in a pan. 4. Serve the chicken with broccoli and almonds. 5. Serve as a tasty main course.

TROUT IN PAPER WITH MIXED VEGETABLES

Preparation time: 20 minutes

Cooking times: 15/20 minutes

Doses for 4 people

Ingredients:

Trout (4 pieces 800 g total)

Mixed vegetables (e.g. courgettes, tomatoes, onion)

Lemon (1)

Fresh parsley

Extra virgin olive oil (60 ml)

Salt and black pepper

Preparation:

1. Stuff the trout with lemon slices, fresh parsley, mixed sliced vegetables, olive oil, salt and pepper. 2. Wrap the trout in baking paper and cook in the oven until cooked. 3. Serve with lemon wedges. 4. Serve as a light and aromatic main course.

BAKED SEA BASS WITH TOMATOES AND OLIVES

Preparation time: 15 minutes

Cooking times: 25/30 minutes

Doses for 4 people

Ingredients:

Sea bass (4 pieces 800 g total)

Cherry tomatoes (200 g)

Black olives (50 g)

Garlic (2 cloves)

Fresh rosemary

Extra virgin olive oil (60 ml)

Salt and black pepper

Preparation:

1. Stuff the 4 pieces of Branzino with cherry tomatoes, black olives, sliced garlic, fresh rosemary, olive oil, salt and pepper. 2. Cook the sea bass in the oven until well cooked and golden. 3. Serve as a fragrant main course.

LEAN MEATBALLS WITH TOMATO SAUCE

Preparation time: 20 minutes

Cooking times: 25/30 minutes

Doses for 4 people

Ingredients:

Lean minced meat (400 g)

Peeled tomatoes (400 g)

Onion (1)

Garlic (2 cloves)

Fresh parsley

Salt and black pepper

Preparation:

1. Mix the lean ground beef with minced garlic, fresh parsley, salt and pepper. Shape into meatballs. 2. Brown the onion and garlic in a pan and add the peeled tomatoes. 3. Cook the meatballs in the tomato sauce until cooked. 4. Serve with fresh parsley as a garnish. 5. Serve as a protein-rich main course.

SOLE WITH LEMON

AND PARSLEY SAUCE

Preparation time: 15 minutes

Cooking times: 10/15 minutes

Doses for 4 people

Ingredients:

4 sole fillets (200 g each)

Lemon (2)

Fresh parsley

Light butter (60 g)

Salt and black pepper

Preparation:

1. Cook the sole fillets in a pan with light butter until golden and cooked through. 2. Make a lemon sauce with lemon juice, grated lemon zest, fresh parsley, salt and pepper. 3. Pour the lemon sauce over the sole fillets. 4. Serve as a light and fragrant main course.

MUSTARD PORK FILLET WITH ASPARAGUS

Preparation time: 20 minutes

Cooking times: 20/25 minutes

Doses for 4 people

Ingredients:

Pork fillet (4 pieces

from 180 g. each)

Dijon mustard (60 g)

Asparagus (400 g)

Garlic (2 cloves)

Fresh rosemary

Salt and black pepper

Preparation:

1. Coat the pork tenderloin with Dijon mustard, minced garlic, fresh rosemary, salt and pepper. 2. Cook the pork tenderloin in the oven until cooked through. 3. Steam the asparagus until tender. 4. Serve the pork fillet with asparagus. 5. Serve as a tasty main course.

CHICKEN CURRY WITH COURGETTES

Preparation time: 20 minutes

Cooking times: 20/25 minutes

Doses for 4 people

Ingredients:

4 chicken breasts (160 g. each)

Courgettes (400 g)

Curry powder (2 tablespoons)

Coconut milk (400 ml)

Onion (1)

Extra virgin olive oil (60 ml)

Salt and black pepper

Preparation:

1. Cut the chicken breast into cubes and brown with chopped onion and olive oil. 2. Add curry powder and cook for a few minutes. 3. Add the diced zucchini and coconut milk. Cook until the courgettes are tender. 4. Complete with salt and pepper. 5. Serve as an aromatic main course.

GRILLED TUNA WITH ARUGULA SALAD

Preparation time: 15 minutes

Cooking times: 5/7 minutes

Doses for 4 people

Ingredients:

4 tuna fillets (180 g. each)

Arugula (200 g)

Lemon (2)

Extra virgin olive oil (60 ml)

Salt and black pepper

Preparation:

1. Marinate the tuna fillet with lemon juice, olive oil, salt and pepper. 2. Heat the grill and cook the tuna until it is golden brown on the outside but still pink on the inside. 3. Serve the tuna with the arugula salad dressed with olive oil and lemon juice. 4. Serve as a light, protein-rich main course.

LAMB SHANK WITH SWEET POTATO PUREE

Preparation time: 20 minutes

Cooking times: 1 hours

Doses for 4 people

Ingredients:

Lamb shank (4 pieces 200 g each)

Sweet potatoes (800 g)

Fresh rosemary

Garlic (2 cloves)

Extra virgin olive oil (60 ml)

Salt and black pepper

Preparation:

1. Brown the lamb shanks with minced garlic and olive oil. 2. Add diced sweet potatoes, fresh rosemary, salt and pepper. 3. Cook in the oven at low temperature until the meat is tender. 4. Make a sweet potato mash with the cooked potatoes and serve with the lamb shanks. 5. Serve as a rustic main course.

ROAST DUCK WITH DRIED PLUM

Preparation time: 15 minutes

Cooking times: 120 minutes

Doses for 4 people

Ingredients:

Duck (1 whole)

Dried plums (150 g)

Onion (1)

Fresh thyme

Salt and black pepper

Preparation:

1. Stuff the duck with prunes, sliced onion, fresh thyme, salt and pepper. 2. Cook the duck in the oven until well roasted and the meat is tender. 3. Serve as a festive main course.

DUCK BREAST IN ORANGE SAUCE

Preparation time: 20 minutes

Cooking times: 15/20 minutes

Doses for 4 people

Ingredients:

Duck breast (4 pieces

from 200 g. each)

Oranges (2)

Honey (60 ml)

Fresh ginger

Salt and black pepper

Preparation:

1. Brown the duck breasts in a pan, skin side down, until the skin is crispy. 2. Cook the duck breasts in the oven until cooked through but still pink inside. 3. Make an orange sauce with orange juice, honey, grated fresh ginger, salt and pepper. 4. Serve the duck breasts with the orange sauce. 5. Serve as an aromatic main course.

VEAL CHOP WITH GRILLED VEGETABLES

Preparation time: 20 minutes

Cooking times: 15/20 minutes

Doses for 4 people

Ingredients:

4 veal chops

(of 200 g. each)

Courgettes (400 g)

Peppers (2)

Eggplant (2)

Extra virgin olive oil (60 ml)

Fresh rosemary

Salt and black pepper

Preparation:

1. Coat the veal chops with olive oil, fresh rosemary, salt and pepper. 2. Grill the veal chops until cooked through and well marked. 3. Grill the courgettes, peppers and sliced aubergines. 4. Serve the veal chops with the grilled vegetables. 5. Serve as a light and tasty main course.

CHICKEN SAUSAGES WITH ROASTED CAULIFLOWER

Preparation time: 20 minutes

Cooking times: 30/35 minutes

Doses for 4 people

Ingredients:

4 chicken sausages (180 g each)

Cauliflowers (1)

Garlic (2 cloves)

Extra virgin olive oil (60 ml)

Fresh rosemary

Salt and black pepper

Preparation:

1. Cook chicken sausages in a pan with minced garlic and olive oil until well cooked. 2. Cut the cauliflower into florets , toss with olive oil, fresh rosemary, salt and pepper, and roast in the oven until golden. 3. Serve the chicken sausages with the roasted cauliflower. 4. Serve as a tasty main course.

SEA BASS FILLET
IN PIECE
WITH FENNEL

Preparation time: 15 minutes

Cooking times: 20/25 minutes

Doses for 4 people

Ingredients:

4 sea bass fillets

(of 180 g. each)

Fennel (2)

Lemon (2)

Fresh thyme

Salt and black pepper

Preparation:

1. Slice the fennel and season it with lemon juice, fresh thyme, salt and pepper. 2. Wrap the sea bass fillets in aluminum foil with the fennel. 3. Cook the parcels in the oven until the fish is cooked. 4. Serve as a light and aromatic main course.

DUCK BREAST WITH BLACK CURRANT SAUCE

Preparation time: 20 minutes

Cooking times: 15/20 minutes

Doses for 4 people

Ingredients:

4 duck breasts (200 g each)

Blackcurrant (200g)

Brown sugar (50 g)

Fresh ginger

Salt and black pepper

Preparation:

1. Brown the duck breasts in a pan until the skin is crispy and the meat is pink inside. 2. Make a blackcurrant sauce with blackcurrants, brown sugar, grated fresh ginger, salt and pepper. 3. Serve the duck breasts with the blackcurrant sauce. 4. Serve as a festive main course.

COCONUT CHICKEN WITH WOKED VEGETABLES

Preparation time: 20 minutes

Cooking times: 15/20 minutes

Doses for 4 people

Ingredients:

Chicken breast (4 pieces from 200 g. each)

Coconut milk (400 ml)

Mixed vegetables for wok (400 g)

Curry powder (2 tablespoons)

Coconut oil (60 ml)

Salt and black pepper

Preparation:

1. Cut the chicken breast into cubes and cook it in a pan with coconut oil. 2. Add vegetables to the wok and cook until tender. 3. Add coconut milk and curry powder. Cook until the chicken is cooked through and the sauce is thick. 4. Complete with salt and pepper. 5. Serve as an exotic main course.

BEEF STEAK WITH GREEN PEPPER

Preparation time: 10 minutes

Cooking times: 10/15 minutes

Doses for 4 people

Ingredients:

Beef steak

(4 pieces of 160 g each)

Fresh cream (200 ml)

Green peppercorns

(2 tablespoons)

Brandy (60ml)

Butter (60 g)

salt

Preparation:

1. Cook the beef steaks in a pan with butter until they are at the desired doneness. 2. Make a green pepper sauce with fresh cream, green peppercorns and brandy. Cook until the sauce is thick. 3. Pour the sauce over the beef steaks. 4. Serve as a succulent main course.

BAKED TROUT WITH ALMONDS

Preparation time: 15 minutes

Cooking times: 20/25 minutes

Doses for 4 people

Ingredients:

4 trout (200 g each)

Almonds (100 g)

Lemon (2)

Butter (60 g)

Fresh parsley

Salt and black pepper

Preparation:

1. Clean the trout and season them with lemon juice, melted butter, salt and pepper. 2. Add sliced almonds on top of the trout. 3. Cook the trout in the oven until cooked through and the almonds are golden. 4. Serve as a light and crunchy main course.

PORK FILLET WITH CRANBERRIES

Preparation time: 15 minutes

Cooking times: 25/30 minutes

Doses for 4 people

Ingredients:

4 pork fillets

(from 200 g each)

Cranberries (150 g)

Balsamic vinegar (60 ml)

Honey (60ml)

Fresh rosemary

Salt and black pepper

Preparation:

1. Brown the pork fillets until golden brown and cooked through . 2. Make cranberry sauce with cranberries, balsamic vinegar, honey, fresh rosemary, salt and pepper. 3. Pour the sauce over the pork tenderloins. 4. Serve as a festive main course.

CHICKEN WITH WALNUTS WITH ARUGULA SALAD

Preparation time: 20 minutes

Cooking times: 20/25 minutes

Doses for 4 people

Ingredients:

Chicken breast (4 pieces

from 200 g. each)

Walnuts (100 g)

Arugula (200 g)

Lemon (2)

Extra virgin olive oil (60 ml)

Salt and black pepper

Preparation:

1. Chop the walnuts finely and sprinkle them on the chicken breasts. 2. Cook the chicken in a pan with olive oil until golden and cooked through. 3. Make a salad with arugula, lemon juice, olive oil, salt and pepper. 4. Serve the chicken with the arugula salad. 5. Serve as a crunchy, protein-rich main course.

LAMB SHANK WITH MINT

Preparation time: 15 minutes

Cooking times: 1 hours

Doses for 4 people

Ingredients:

4 lamb shanks

(from 180 g. each)

Fresh mint

Garlic (2 cloves)

Extra virgin olive oil (60 ml)

Salt and black pepper

Preparation:

1. Brown the lamb shanks with minced garlic and olive oil. 2. Add fresh mint leaves, salt and pepper. 3. Cook in the oven at low temperature until the meat is tender. 4. Serve as a rustic main course.

SALMON IN PISTACHIO CRUST

Preparation time: 15 minutes

Cooking times: 15/20 minutes

Doses for 4 people

Ingredients:

4 salmon fillets

(from 200 g each)

Chopped pistachios (100 g)

Lemon (2)

Butter (60 g)

Fresh parsley

Salt and black pepper

Preparation:

1. Mix chopped pistachios with melted butter, grated lemon zest, fresh parsley, salt and pepper. 2. Spread this mixture on the salmon fillets. 3. Bake until the salmon is cooked through and the crust is golden brown. 4. Serve as a crunchy and tasty main course.

VEAL CUTLETS
MILANESE STYLE

Preparation time: 20 minutes

Cooking times: 10/15 minutes

Doses for 4 people

Ingredients:

4 veal cutlets

(from 220 g. each)

Grated bread (150 g)

Eggs (2)

Grated parmesan (50 g)

Lemon (2)

Butter (60 g)

Salt and black pepper

Preparation:

1. Dip the veal chops in beaten eggs and breadcrumbs mixed with grated parmesan. 2. Cook the ribs in a pan with butter until golden and crispy. 3. Top with lemon slices. 4. Serve as a crunchy and tasty main course.

CHICKEN CURRY WITH SPINACH

Preparation time: 20 minutes

Cooking times: 20/25 minutes

Doses for 4 people

Ingredients:

4 chicken breasts

(from 180 g. each)

Fresh spinach (400 g)

Coconut milk (400 ml)

Curry powder (2 tablespoons)

Extra virgin olive oil (60 ml)

Salt and black pepper

Preparation:

1. Cook the chicken in a pan with olive oil until golden and cooked through. 2. Add fresh spinach and cook until wilted. 3. Pour in the coconut milk and curry powder. Cook until the chicken is cooked through and the sauce is thick. 4. Complete with salt and pepper. 5. Serve as a main course full of flavour.

BEEF STEAK
WITH ROSEMARY

Preparation time: 10 minutes

Cooking times: 10/15 minutes

Doses for 4 people

Ingredients:

Beef steak

(4 pieces of 200 g each)

Fresh rosemary

Garlic (2 cloves)

Extra virgin olive oil (60 ml)

Salt and black pepper

Preparation:

1. Brown beef steaks with fresh rosemary, minced garlic and olive oil until desired doneness. 2. Complete with salt and pepper. 3. Serve as a rustic and aromatic main course.

MEDITERRANEAN STYLE COD

Preparation time: 15 minutes

Cooking times: 20/25 minutes

Doses for 4 people

Ingredients:

4 cod fillets

(of 160 g. each)

Tomatoes (4)

Black olives (100 g)

Capers (2 tablespoons)

Dried oregano

Extra virgin olive oil (60 ml)

Salt and black pepper

Preparation:

1. Place the cod fillets on a baking tray. 2. Add sliced tomatoes, black olives, capers, oregano, olive oil, salt and pepper. 3. Bake until the fish is cooked and the tomatoes are soft. 4. Serve as a light, Mediterranean-flavored main course.

DUCK IN PLUM SAUCE

Preparation time: 20 minutes

Cooking times: 1/42 hours

Doses for 4 people

Ingredients:

Duck breast (4 pieces)

Dried plums (200 g)

Fresh ginger

Garlic (2 cloves)

Red wine (200 ml)

Honey (60 ml)

Salt and black pepper

Preparation:

1. Brown the duck breasts in a pan with minced garlic and fresh ginger until golden brown. 2. Add prunes, red wine, honey, salt and pepper. 3. Cook over low heat until the duck is tender and the sauce is thick. 4. Serve as a rich, festive main course.

SWEET AND SOUR PORK WITH PEPPERS

Preparation time: 20 minutes

Cooking times: 20/25 minutes

Doses for 4 people

Ingredients:

Diced pork (400 g)

Peppers (2)

Onion (1)

Wine vinegar (60 ml)

Sugar (60 g)

Soy sauce (60 ml)

Extra virgin olive oil (60 ml)

Salt and black pepper

Preparation:

1. Brown the pork in a pan with olive oil until browned. 2. Add striped peppers, sliced onion, wine vinegar, sugar and soy sauce. 3. Cook until the pork is cooked through and the sauce is thick. 4. Complete with salt and pepper. 5. Serve as a sweet and sour main course.

CHICKEN BREAST WITH MUSTARD

Preparation time: 15 minutes

Cooking times: 20/25 minutes

Doses for 4 people

Ingredients:

4 chicken breasts

(from 200 g each)

Dijon mustard (4 tablespoons)

Honey (4 tablespoons)

Fresh rosemary

Extra virgin olive oil (60 ml)

Salt and black pepper

Preparation:

1. Spread Dijon mustard and honey over chicken breasts. 2. Cook the chicken in a pan with olive oil until golden and cooked through. 3. Add fresh rosemary leaves, salt and pepper. 4. Serve as a main course with a robust flavor.

SALMON WITH SAUCE
OF LEMON AND DILL

Preparation time: 15 minutes

Cooking times: 1520 minutes

Doses for 4 people

Ingredients:

4 salmon fillets

(160 g. each)

Lemon (2)

Fresh dill

Butter (60 g)

Salt and black pepper

Preparation:

1. Cook the salmon fillets in a pan with butter until golden and cooked through. 2. Make a sauce with lemon juice, fresh dill, salt and pepper. 3. Pour the sauce over the salmon fillets. 4. Serve as a fresh and fragrant main course.

GRILLED VEGETABLES

Preparation time: 15 minutes

Cooking time: 20 minutes

Dose for: 2 people

Ingredients

1 courgette

1 aubergine

1 red pepper

1 yellow pepper

100 g of champignon mushrooms

2 tablespoons extra virgin olive oil

1 clove of garlic

Aromatic herbs (rosemary,

thyme, oregano) to taste Salt to taste Pepper to taste

Preparation

1 Prepare the ingredients: Wash all the vegetables well. Cut the courgette and aubergine into slices about 1 cm thick. Cut the peppers in half, remove the seeds and cut into wide strips. Clean the mushrooms by removing the lower part of the stem and leaving them whole if they are small, or cutting them in half if they are large. Finely chop the garlic. 2. Season the vegetables: In a large bowl, place all the cut vegetables. Add the olive oil, minced garlic, herbs, salt and pepper. Mix well to make sure all the vegetables are well seasoned. 3. Grill the vegetables: Preheat the grill to medium-high heat . Arrange the vegetables on the grill in a single layer. Cook for about 10 minutes per side, or until the vegetables are tender and lightly charred. 4. Serve: Remove the vegetables from the grill and arrange them on a serving platter. Serve hot, accompanied by a drizzle of olive oil

BAKED POTATOES

Preparation time: 10 minutes

Cooking time: 40 minutes

Dose for: 2 people

Ingredients

4 medium potatoes

2 tablespoons of oil

extra virgin olive oil

1 sprig of fresh rosemary

2 cloves of garlic

Salt to taste Pepper to taste

Preparation

1. Prepare the ingredients: Preheat the oven to 200°C. Wash the potatoes well and, if you prefer, peel them. Cut them into cubes of approximately 23 cm. Finely chop the garlic cloves. Wash the rosemary sprig and remove the leaves from the stems. 2. Season the potatoes: In a large bowl, place the cut potatoes. Add the olive oil, minced garlic, rosemary leaves, salt and pepper. Mix well to make sure all the potatoes are well seasoned. 3. Cook the potatoes: Arrange the seasoned potatoes in a single layer on a baking sheet. Bake in the preheated oven for about 40 minutes, or until the potatoes are golden brown and crispy on the outside and tender on the inside. Stir the potatoes halfway through cooking for even browning. 4. Serve: Remove the potatoes from the oven and transfer them to a serving plate. Serve hot, perhaps accompanied by a drizzle of extra virgin olive oil and a sprinkling of fresh rosemary.

SAUTEED SPINACH

Preparation time: 5 minutes

Cooking time: 5 minutes

Dose for: 2 people

Ingredients

300 g of fresh spinach

2 tablespoons of oil

extra virgin olive oil

2 cloves of garlic

Salt to taste Pepper to taste

Lemon juice (optional)

Preparation

1. Prepare the ingredients: Wash the spinach well and dry it. Peel and finely slice the garlic cloves. 2. Saute the spinach: In a large skillet, heat the olive oil over medium heat.

Add the sliced garlic and sauté until golden, being careful not to burn it. Add the spinach to the pan. Cook, stirring constantly, until the spinach is wilted and tender, about 35 minutes. Season with salt and pepper to taste. 3. Serve: Transfer the sautéed spinach to a serving platter. Add a squeeze of lemon juice, if desired, for a touch of freshness. Serve immediately as a side dish

SAUTÉED MUSHROOMS

Preparation time: 10 minutes

Cooking time: 15 minutes

Dose for: 2 people

Ingredients

300 g of fresh champignon mushrooms

2 tablespoons of oil

extra virgin olive oil

2 cloves of garlic

1 bunch of fresh parsley

Salt to taste Pepper to taste

Preparation

1. Prepare the ingredients: Clean the mushrooms with a damp cloth or kitchen brush to remove any residual soil.

Cut the mushrooms into slices. Peel and finely chop the garlic cloves. Finely chop the parsley. 2. Cook the mushrooms: In a large skillet, heat the olive oil over medium heat. Add the chopped garlic and sauté until golden, being careful not to burn it. Add the sliced mushrooms to the pan. Cook, stirring occasionally, until the mushrooms release their water and are tender and lightly browned, about 1015 minutes. Season with salt and pepper to taste. 3. Add the parsley: Just before finishing cooking, add the chopped parsley and mix well. 4. Serve: Transfer the sautéed mushrooms to a serving plate. Serve hot as a side dish.

STEAMED BROCCOLI

Preparation time: 5 minutes

Cooking time: 10 minutes

Dose for: 2 people

Ingredients

1 medium broccoli

2 tablespoons of oil

extra virgin olive oil

1 clove of garlic (optional)

Juice of half a lemon

Salt to taste Pepper to taste

Preparation

1. Prepare the ingredients: Wash the broccoli well and cut it into florets . If desired, peel and finely chop the garlic. 2. Steam: Fill a pot with about 23cm of water and bring it to the boil. Place the broccoli in a steamer basket and place it over the pot of boiling water. Cover with a lid. Steam the broccoli for about 810 minutes, or until tender but still crunchy . 3. Season the broccoli: Transfer the cooked broccoli to a bowl. Add the olive oil, lemon juice, salt and pepper. If using, also add minced garlic. Mix well to make sure the broccoli is well seasoned. 4. Serve: Transfer the steamed broccoli to a serving platter. Serve immediately as a side dish

CONCLUSION

Conclusion: Embracing a Future of Health and Wellness As we come to the end of our journey through the Dissociated Diet 2025, I hope you have found inspiration, knowledge, and a new perspective on your nutrition and health. This book was created to help you discover a balanced and fulfilling way of eating that allows you to achieve your weight loss goals, but goes beyond, promoting healthier living and lasting well-being. You've learned how to combine foods intelligently to optimize your nutritional intake, while enjoying delicious, nutritious meals. Your opinion matters If you found this book useful, we kindly invite you to leave a review.

The 120 recipes presented in this book have been carefully selected to offer you a variety of flavors and options, allowing you to maintain your motivation in your quest for a healthier life. In addition to the recipes, you have gained a scientific understanding of the Dissociated Diet and its basic principles. This approach aims to make you feel in control of your food choices and how they affect your health. The practical advice provided will help you plan balanced meals and maintain your commitment to a healthier life. The key to success with the Dissociated Diet 2025 is perseverance and awareness. Continue to experiment with recipes, explore new ways of cooking, and maintain an active lifestyle.

Remember that wellness is an ongoing journey, and every step you take toward a balanced diet and a healthy body is a step toward your future of health and wellness. Today you took control of your diet and your life. Now, with the tools and knowledge you have acquired, you are ready to embrace a future where health, well-being and the pleasure of eating come together in a symphony of happiness. Thank you for choosing the Dissociated Diet 2025 to guide you on your journey to a healthier, happier you . Adopting the Dissociated Diet is a commitment to a healthier lifestyle, based on an in-depth understanding of food combinations and their effects on our body.

We are happy to have accompanied you on this journey towards a personalized and healthy diet. We hope the recipes and information in this book have inspired you to make more conscious food choices and achieve your wellness goals.

Whether you are new to the Dissociated Diet , or an expert, we hope that the "Dissociated Diet 2025 has been a valuable ally on your path to a healthier and more fulfilling life.

We wish you bon appetit and a future radiant with health and happiness!

Sincerely, [KLARLOCK]

www.ingramcontent.com/pod-product-compliance
Lightning Source LLC
Chambersburg PA
CBHW061922270726
48659CB00001BA/93